SILVER LININGS

Surviving Breast Cancer

SILVER LININGS

Surviving Breast Cancer

M J Ebdell

ATHENA PRESS
LONDON

SILVER LININGS
Surviving Breast Cancer
Copyright © M J Ebdell 2007

ISBN 10-digit: 1 84401 898 9
ISBN 13-digit: 978 1 84401 898 7

First Published 2007 by
ATHENA PRESS
Queen's House, 2 Holly Road
Twickenham TW1 4EG
United Kingdom

Printed for Athena Press

Part One

What Happened First

This photograph was taken in Kenya, in December 2004, before anything was wrong. Two months later my hair was even longer. I was doing it myself using longer extensions. The braids reached my waist and many of them were finished off with beads. Everyone said how well it suited me and I loved it.

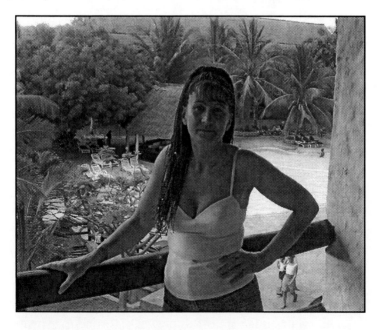

Life was good then. I thought the world was a wonderful place and felt lucky that my family could share it with me. But in April 2005, I heard the words no one ever wants to hear: 'I'm sorry. But you have cancer.'

I first realised that breast cancer can affect women of any age about twenty years ago and, from that moment on, I decided to check myself regularly. At first it was just when I remembered, as I got into the shower in the mornings. Then it got to be about once a week. Soon it became an everyday habit. And every day I would find nothing unusual, until one day in February 2005.

That morning everything had been fine, but in the evening, as I undressed for another shower, I noticed something strange. I was forty-four years old, and had given birth to two little boys. My boobs were no longer 'pert' by any stretch of the imagination. But, as I took off the scaffolding that M&S sold as a bra, only one of my boobs drooped. The left one stayed exactly where it was – pert and hard!

It was a Friday evening so I decided that if it was still hard on Monday then I would make an appointment with my GP.

On the Monday morning I made the phone call, but it wasn't as easy as it sounds. At my doctor's practice I had to ring between eight and eight thirty in the morning to make an appointment for that day, but it was almost nine thirty before I finally managed to get through. It was too late for that day and they didn't make appointments in advance. I would have to try again the next day.

This went on for almost three weeks. I tried to explain to the receptionist that I had lumps in my breast and, by then, under my arm as well, I was just told, 'I'm sorry, there's nothing I can do. It's Tony Blair's new plan.'

I was convinced I had cancer. It wasn't just the rock hard boob and the lumps under my arm, it was also the weight gain that I couldn't shift, and a feeling in my heart. I just knew.

Eventually I did manage to get an appointment to see my GP.

'It's hormonal,' she said, 'nothing to worry about.'

I told her that I had been 'hormonal' for over thirty years and this had never happened before, but she didn't seem to hear. 'Come back in two weeks' time,' she told me. 'It'll be gone by then.' I pointed out that it had already been there for three weeks and asked what the lumps under my arm were, but she simply repeated that I should come back in two weeks' time and it would be gone.

If she hadn't been heavily pregnant I think I might have said more. I wanted to hit her! But I didn't say what I thought it was. I just couldn't get the words out of my mouth. I had learnt that as long as I never actually said the word 'cancer' then I could cope. I desperately wanted to believe this woman, who was supposed to know about these things. I did as she said and began trying to make another appointment almost immediately. It took another three weeks.

'Oh, hasn't it gone then?' she asked.

'No, and the lumps under my arm are so big now that I can't hold my arm straight down any more. I want to see a specialist.' That was as close as I could get to admitting what I thought was wrong.

Eventually, she relented and told me, 'I'll write a letter, but it will be a long wait I'm afraid. After all, it's not important.'

I got my appointment for five weeks later. While I was waiting, I noticed one of those mobile breast-screening units in Tesco's car park. I already knew what was wrong with me, but I needed someone to notice. So I went in. But I wasn't allowed to have a mammogram. I was told, 'If your GP says it's nothing, then it's nothing.'

I was also told, 'My dear, you are far too young to have breast cancer!' Stupid woman, if I could find her now I would shove her head in that mammogram machine and squash it!

I got a letter asking me to go in for two types of test on the same day as my appointment. The test would be first and then I would meet Mr Laidlaw.

There is no way the specialist could possibly have any idea what the results of those test would be when I saw him that afternoon in April. I sat on the bed behind the curtain after stripping off my shirt and bra. Mr Laidlaw came in and looked at me. Then he poked and prodded both my breasts and told me to get dressed. A few minutes later, as my husband Rob and I sat by the man's desk he told us, 'I'm very sorry, but I'm ninety-nine per cent certain that you have cancer.' I didn't hear what else he said. I just hated him.

The next few weeks were a constant round of trips to Frimley Park Hospital and St Luke's Cancer Centre in Guildford. I was poked and prodded and I was tested. I had things shoved into me and bits cut out of me. I went under machines and through machines and was even nuked! Well, someone from 'Nuclear Medicine' came and shoved something into my arm. 'Great,' I said, 'I spend ten years trying to be chemical free and now you go and nuke me!' The guy laughed.

It was while waiting for one of my appointments at St Luke's that I spotted a familiar hairdo on top of a familiar pair of shoulders. 'Sue?' I said, and she turned around. 'What are you doing here?' I didn't know Sue very well at that point, she was just 'that happy woman from Homestart' (Homestart was in the same community centre as the on-line centre where I worked). I had no idea that she had cancer. She told me it was in her chest and that she was being treated by taking chemo tablets. She smiled as she told me that she wasn't going to lose her hair this time. This time? So she'd had it before then! Very quickly after that Sue became to me just what she was to so many other people in her job as a care worker. She became someone I could talk to; someone who understood what I was going through; someone to make me laugh and tell me everything was going to be just fine.

Then I found myself back at that desk in front of Mr Laidlaw. Rob said he had a beard at that point, but I wouldn't know, I couldn't look at him. I hated him.

That day he talked about 'controlling' my cancer and he explained about the chemo I would need. He then said that he was sorry, but I would lose my hair. I hated him even more then. Then another doctor came into the room. She had something quite important to tell me. After faffing about trying to find the right words, she finally told me, 'I'm really sorry, but, er, the chemo will, er, I'm afraid, um, affect your fertility. I'm so sorry, but there's very little chance you will be able to have any more children.'

The poor woman had gone through so much to get

those words out, I had to put her feelings at ease. 'Thank heavens for that!' I said – much to her surprise. 'I'm forty-four, I've got polycystic ovaries, blocked tubes and a son about to hit his teens. If you can get rid of that monthly problem for me it would be great!'

She then told me that my 'monthly problem' would disappear. So there was my first silver lining. Freedom! Well, if you're not having any more kids, what on earth do you want *that* for?

That night I made a decision. If I was going to lose my long hair, then it was going to be on *my* terms. The next day I went over to the wig shop in Sandhurst and had all my hair cut off.

'Are you sure?' asked the woman.

'Yes.'

It was done very well. Two women were there. It would have been much easier for them if just one of them had started to cut from the top and worked down, but instead one woman held up my braids as the other began snipping from the back. They kept me talking and didn't really give me time for more than a few small tears. When it was all off, they asked if I wanted to keep the braids. I said no and was immediately whisked off into another room to have what was left washed. I never saw the braids.

I then spent the next two or three hours trying on wigs. No matter how many I wanted to try, or how many times I changed my mind, the two women didn't mind. Even when I ended up with the very first one I had been shown no one complained. It cost just under £300 and Robert didn't mind either. I later discovered that the fancy dress shop in Aldershot sold really good wigs for just £30. I bought a blond one and it looked real. My friend Mandy once asked me, 'Can you text before you come over again and let me know what colour your hair is, I never know who to look out for.' Another good friend who lives in America sent me a bright blue wig, complete with brightly coloured ribbons. That caused a bit of a stir at the school when I wore it to meet Billy. Fortunately my son has a fantastic sense of humour, but some of the mothers thought I was round the twist!

However, the first day I wore a wig I was nervous about going to the school to fetch Billy. Some mothers waiting outside the school gates can be scary. I knew that everyone would wonder why I'd lost the braids and I was convinced they would see straight away that I was wearing a wig. I knew they would want to know why, but that they would never ask. Instead they were likely to make up their own minds. I didn't want to walk through that gate alone if I was going to be stared at, so I called on Mandy and Clair for support.

They were waiting on the pavement as I drove the van around the corner and parked. Clair could hardly believe the hair. 'It's fantastic,' she said. And she sounded as if she meant it, which made me feel good. Mandy was also convinced that no one would guess it wasn't real hair and the three of us walked into the school together. I did get a few strange looks, but with Mandy on my left and Clair on my right, both acting as daft as usual, I didn't care.

Billy's face was a picture when he saw me. His eyes went so wide I thought they might pop out of his head, but he soon regained composure, dropped his bag at my feet and asked, 'Can I have some money to go to the shop?'

Mandy and Clair's children did not get told about my wig until some time later and, in the meantime, they just treated me as normal. I don't think they even noticed.

Then I found myself sitting in Dr Laing's room at St Luke's again.

'I want you to try the cold cap,' he said. Apparently this is a kind of frozen motorcycle helmet that is worn for two hours before chemo and about three hours afterwards. The idea is that it freezes the scalp and saves the hair. Freeze the scalp! It sounded awful. Sue had already told me how my hair would probably grow back thicker and stronger and may even be curly, so why would I want to freeze my scalp just to keep the pin-straight, thin hair I had before?

'Oh, no. It doesn't matter about the hair,' I said.

'But hair like that! You really should think about saving it,' he said.

'It really doesn't matter,' I insisted as I grabbed my fringe and pulled off my hair. His face was a picture! Either he really had thought it was real hair, or he was one hell of an actor!

That same day, I was meant to get the results of all the tests I had taken, but they weren't there. 'I'll chase them up' said Dr Laing, and off he went.

Rob and I sat there in silence until I said, 'We're sitting here waiting to hear if I'm going to live or die.'

Then the door opened again and Dr Laing's head appeared around it. 'Got them,' he said. 'They are all clear.' He then grinned and disappeared. That meant the cancer was only in my left breast, not anywhere else. There was a chance I was going to live through this after all.

The next thing to happen was that I had a line fitted. This was a small plastic tube that entered my chest just between my cleavage. It travelled under my skin to a point just by my right collarbone. Then it entered a vein and headed off towards my heart. This was how the chemo would be administered. The tube hung out from my chest to just above my waist. At the end was a bung to connect to the pump I would need to wear.

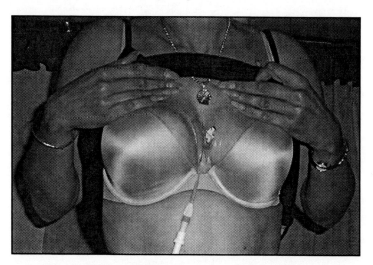

It was the day after the line was fitted that I discovered my wig had been noticed, and discussed, by several mothers as they waited outside the school gates. Mandy told me about it first and said that she was sorry but she had told them about my cancer to shut them up. I heard the full story from someone else.

The mothers' conversation went something like this:

'It's got to be a wig, it's better than her own hair ever was.'

'Of course it's a wig, those braids would have ruined her own hair.'

'Why doesn't she just admit she ruined it and have it short?'

'Maybe it damaged her scalp!'

And that was when Mandy had apparently heard enough. Steaming into this small group with a face that said she meant business she shouted, 'You don't have to stand there making up your own minds because I'll tell you the truth – yes, it is a wig, but she didn't ruin her hair, she's got bloody cancer!' She then turned and calmly walked to the relevant classroom to fetch her daughter, leaving the others feeling rather small and looking as if they had just been slapped!

Part Two
Chemo

So then the chemo started. My appointment at St Luke's would usually be for about two o'clock in the afternoon. So I would have to be there by about twelve. I had to have a blood test done first to check to see if I was well enough for the chemo.

Then I would see the doctor. It wasn't always Dr Laing, often one of his team. They were a bunch of really nice people. I particularly liked one African doctor. I can't remember his name, but he really gave the impression that he hated to see people ill. You could just see it in his face as he thought, Oh no, someone is ill, I must make them better.

After this I would finally be hooked up to the chemical that would, hopefully, shrink my lumps to a size small enough to be removed.

I think there were actually two types of chemical that were pumped into the line in my chest. Then there were the steroids to go in and the bone drug. This drug was new and is still being tested. They claimed that it didn't have any side effects at all, but they were not sure how well it worked. So only three thousand of us worldwide were allowed to have it. (Apparently.)

You see, it is believed that chemotherapy can cause osteoporosis and this drug was designed to prevent that. I would need to have it every three months for five years before they could tell if it worked.

After all this there was the pump. That was attached to the bung at the end of my line and would drip chemo into my heart twenty-four hours a day, seven days a week. Not pleasant!

I would have to have that changed every week. At first I went to St Luke's every Tuesday, but soon I convinced them to teach me to change it myself. I'm glad I did because I soon became too ill to drive.

'Hide it in your clothing,' one nurse told me that first day. 'Pop it down your trouser leg.' Excuse me! The thing was nine inches long and four inches wide. How was I going to 'hide' that in anything? Even if I could have got it down the leg of my jeans it was going to make a few men jealous! I tried pinning it to my bra under my arm, but it just got in the way. If I pinned it to my waistband, it jabbed into my leg when I sat down. In the end I bought a bum bag and put it in there. It would just have to sit on my waist for the next six months.

At first, things weren't too bad. I remember feeling hot and sometimes sick if I stayed out in the sun, but that was about it. When I started to feel sick later on I just drank a fizzy drink to stop it. I'm not sure why, but somehow fizzy drinks seem to stop nausea. I had been given loads of anti-sickness pills, but I never took them. My nails grew too, really fast and long. I wore my wig and felt that I looked quite good, until the sun came out.

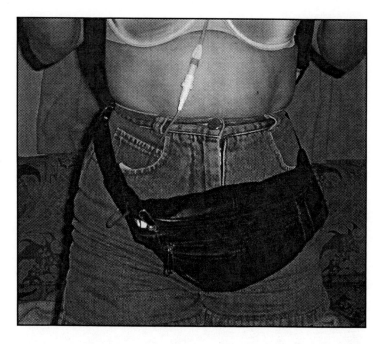

One day I sat with friends at a campsite in Laleham. The wig was making me so hot that sweat was running down my face. 'Get up,' said Margie. 'You and I are going shopping for a head scarf.' I didn't seem to have a choice in the matter, so off we went to Staines.

I didn't like any of the scarves we saw. I didn't want to look like a cancer victim. So I bought two long scarves from an Indian shop. There were tassels on the ends of them. When I got them home I cut them in half and stitched up the ends, making two squares out of each, with tassels on one side. I didn't realise that you are meant to fold the squares into a triangle, so I just took one end, wrapped it around my head and tied it at the back. The end with the tassels on hung down my back and everyone said it looked really good. So that's what I wore for the next few months and the next time I put on a wig it was for a friend's party. I then realised just how ill I was. I looked as if I had already died! So I went back to using the scarves.

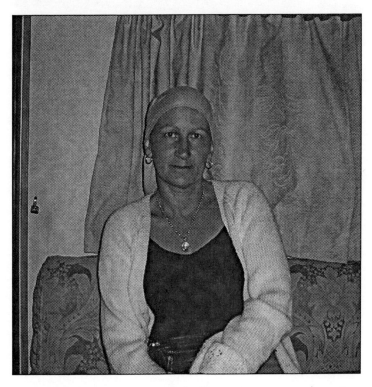

At least this way I only looked old, and not ill.

I was afraid that everyone could see I had cancer if I looked ill, but on the day that I met the brother of a friend of a friend's sister's cousin (or something like that) I realised that maybe I did just look old.

I was sitting in my friend's garden enjoying the sun and sipping a cider when the moron walked in. Everyone knows a moron like this: tall and skinny, doesn't shave very often, hardly washes, never changes his clothes (probably sleeps in them too), and smells of smoke, cheep booze and BO. He stared at me for a while, then blinked and shook his head, tripped over the biscuit tin and sat on the edge of the compost heap. I winked at him and saw the fear spread across his face.

For a while he was silent. Well, at least I assume he was – certainly no one was paying him any attention. Then I heard, 'No I don't want a f—ing cup of tea. I want a f—ing beer!' and, without meaning to, I turned and looked in his direction. That was when he struggled to his feet and staggered towards me with his hand out in front of him. When the hand, palm up, was almost under my nose he opened his mouth and I almost choked on the stench of his halitosis.

'Read my palm,' he demanded, waving his hand about. 'Go on, if you're a gypsy, read my palm.'

'I don't read palms,' I told him, 'but I can tell you your future.'

'Oh yeah?'

'Yeah! If you don't get your hand away from my face, I'm going to put my fist in yours!'

It wasn't just the hair on my head that fell out. I don't understand why people don't realise this, but it's *all* hair. Even those fine hairs on the face. At first this was nice: a whole summer without shaving my bikini line or my legs; a whole summer without shaving under my arms. Another silver lining.

Losing 'other' hair was not so nice. I don't know how little girls cope. I felt really hot and uncomfortable. And when my nose started to run constantly I realised the hairs up there had gone too.

I soon learnt to hate going to St Luke's. It's a good place to be treated and the people are all really nice, but it's the thought of the chemo that everyone hates. And the wait!

First you have the blood test and you wait for the results. Then you wait to see the doctor and, after that, you wait for the chemo. Often it was seven o'clock in the evening before we got out of there. It wasn't anyone's fault, it's just that they were so busy. The nurses don't sit about or waste time, they sort of 'speed walk' everywhere and usually do at least two things at once. I even saw one nurse holding the phone in her left hand and speaking into it while writing out a blood form for someone else with her right hand, but that waiting was so depressing, especially when I just wanted to get it over with and get out of there.

Sometimes, if the wait seemed too long and I had read all the magazines, and if there was no one to talk to (some people chat away and laugh about their condition, but others just don't want to communicate at all), I would wander off and find a nurse.

'How many people are waiting ahead of me?' I would ask.

If I was next in line I would simply sit down again, but often I was told, 'Don't worry, there's two others before you, you've got time for some fresh air,' and I would head out of the door for a smoke.

I know the entrance to the cancer unit isn't the best place to smoke, but loads of us were smokers so we all agreed that this was the wrong time to give it up. Once

I saw a woman in a wheelchair puffing away. Between coughs and splutters she asked me where my cancer was.

'Left boob,' I answered. 'Where's yours?'

Cough, cough. 'Lungs,' cough, splutter, puff! She made the rest of us feel a lot better!

I tried to carry on as normal most of the time, but slowly things changed. Slowly, Rob took over more and more of the things I usually did and Nipper (our funny little dog) learnt that he could no longer jump up at me. I love dogs and there were several that Nipper and I would meet in the park in the mornings. Some of these dogs knew that I was happy to be greeted by them jumping up for some affection, but now they had to learn not to do that. With that line poking out of the bottom of my t-shirt I just couldn't risk it. The last thing I wanted was to have that thing ripped out of my chest by a stray claw! Most of them learnt fast, as long as they still got their ears tickled. Only Keko caused me a slight problem. It wasn't her fault, she is a lovely, friendly, extremely healthy Rottweiler, and she was only playing, but she's several stone of sheer muscle. If you get in her way while she's playing chase – well, it's going to hurt, but once again I got lucky.

When Keko had ploughed into her owner, Lisa, she really had done it well. Lisa did a flying starfish and ended up sprawled face down in the mud. When Keko hit me, she did it from behind and just kept going. It was as if, to her, my legs didn't exist, but, of course, they did. As this huge dog tried to run under me my legs were thrown up into the air in front of me at a perfect right angle to the rest of my body. Then, when my body had had time to register that the legs were no longer underneath me, I sat down. It was actually quite elegantly done. And at least I didn't have my face in the mud or my pump pulled, pushed or yanked. I sat there on the grass and watched as Keko bounded around the park after Nipper and I asked Lisa not to tell her off. The dogs were so happy; I just couldn't spoil their fun.

Then the mouth ulcers came. I'm not talking little pinprick sized things that cause moderate amounts of pain. I'm talking about inch long slugs that roam around the mouth and settle in the throat preventing easy breathing and swallowing. We were staying with my brother Stephen when the ulcers first showed themselves. His girlfriend, Evelyn, had cooked a wonderful roast dinner. It looked and smelt lovely, but I just sat and cried because I couldn't eat anything. The only thing I could drink was iced water and the only thing I could eat was ice cream.

By the time we got back to Surrey and St Luke's was open again I couldn't even swallow water. I walked into St Luke's with a pen and paper in my hand and wrote out a note for the receptionist.

'Could I please see a doctor,' it said. 'My ulcers are so bad that I cannot eat or talk.' I was told to find a chair and wait.

I had taken a book with me. I had seen how busy St Luke's can get and thought I was in for a long wait, but just five minutes after I had sat down the lovely African doctor came out to find me. When he looked into my mouth I could see he was horrified.

'My word, you can't live like that!' he said, and proceeded to write out prescriptions for several different mouthwashes and pills as well as drinks to have instead of food. He asked how I was feeling apart from the ulcers and I said OK. So he gave me one of his 'I know better' looks and I admitted that I was tired a lot. I communicated this with a few grunts, a couple of nods, and closing my eyes. He told me to come back at any time at all if I felt I needed help. I was not to just feel ill and ignore it.

Everyone I met at St Luke's was this nice, from the receptionists to the doctors to the cleaners. Everyone was lovely. I even had a laugh sometimes with the nurses who administered the chemo. I guess they have to be special people to work with cancer patients, but I think St Luke's has got the best of the best.

My mouth ulcers soon began to shrink and drop off. Yes, I said drop off. They didn't just disappear; they dried up and dropped off. Highly unpleasant!

The last to go was the one in my throat. I could feel that it was dying and drying out, but it remained attached to one side of my throat for several days. I could feel it move as I talked or swallowed. It kept making me sick.

Then I started to get really ill.

One day I picked Billy up from school in our motor home and felt so bad that I just drove to the Laleham campsite and booked us in. Then I went to bed.

A couple of days later Billy realised that I had been asleep for more than forty-eight hours, only waking up when he had made me a drink or something to eat.

None of which I kept down. I came out of a troubled sleep to hear him on the phone to his dad. 'I think you'd better come home,' he was saying, 'Mum needs to go to hospital.'

St Peter's in Chertsey would have been nearer, but I wanted to go to the Royal Surrey Hospital. St Luke's is a wing connected to that hospital and I knew the cancer ward was just around the corner from where I saw Dr Laing and had my chemo. I felt I would be better off at a place where the people knew me and knew how to treat me. I wanted to be with familiar faces and people I knew I could trust.

I was in the isolation ward for about a week, but I don't remember much about it. I was in bed asleep most of the time with a drip.

I know that the drip was changed several times a day. There were two types of stuff going into my body. One was, of course, to keep me fed as I couldn't eat, and one was full of heavy-duty antibiotics. The pump was removed at this point and left off for two weeks to allow me to recover.

By then my hands and feet were burning too. That is the only way I can describe it. It was as if I had walked barefoot over hot coals and then held them in my hands. Apart from being a little swollen, my hands and feet looked fine, but the nurses knew they were far from it. I couldn't even touch the sheet on my bed. I had to be washed. Had I been able to swallow I would have had to be fed as well.

Anyone coming into my room had to scrub up first and put on gloves and a gown. Everyone did this except the cleaner, but then she wiped the toilet, sink and windowsill with the same cloth, in that order, and called the room clean. So I can't really expect her to worry about cleaning herself for my health, can I?

Once I was taken for an X-ray. I was given a mask to wear over my face and helped into a wheelchair and then I was taken to another part of the hospital. I have a friend who works at the Royal Surrey and I spent the whole of the trip with my head down praying that it would be his day off. But when I got back to my room I caught sight of myself in the mirror, I needn't have worried, there was no way Carl would have associated this bald, grey-faced old woman with the bouncy, tanned redhead he often trained with at martial arts. I thought of the class, just about a mile down the road from where I was. All those people with all that energy. I made up my mind that I was going to be one of them again just as soon as possible.

One night, towards the end of my stay, I was watching telly when an advert for food came on. There was this lovely, juicy sirloin steak; all pink in the middle, and with loads of chips on the side. My favourite meal (it was just missing the egg). But I hadn't been able to eat anything for days. I admit I cried. A short while later a new nurse came into my room. He introduced himself and told me that he really worked in London and only came to the Royal Surrey when they were short-staffed.

'How are you feeling?' he asked.

'I'm feeling a bit sorry for myself,' I replied, 'but I know I shouldn't. I know there are a lot of people a lot worse off than me.'

'You have a right to feel sorry for yourself, but you are right, there are a lot of people worse off than you,' he said. He then told me that he worked with the terminally ill in London. I wondered about the people he was talking about, how it would feel to know you were dying. I have since been told that I came close to it, but I was never in any doubt that I would recover. Lying there in that bed that night, not able to get up or even to eat or drink, I felt very grateful.

The worst thing about that week in hospital was that it was also the time my dad was over from his home in Tenerife. He was meant to come and visit us, but had to stay with my brother instead. I was too ill to see him.

I then had a free week. That meant that after I got out of the hospital I didn't have the pump put back on for another few days. I spent those days in the sun at the Laleham campsite, and I spent a lot of time hiding from Sandra too. This deputy warden for the site knew the effect the sun could have on someone on chemo and would often yell at me 'You'll get sick' or 'Your skin will get damaged' and she would shove me back into the shade, just before she asked if there was anything I wanted from the shop!

By now my hands and feet were showing the signs of having been burnt. The pain had all gone, but now the blisters came. At first it was just small parts of the palms of my hands and the soles of my feet.

At first it just 'didn't look very nice'.

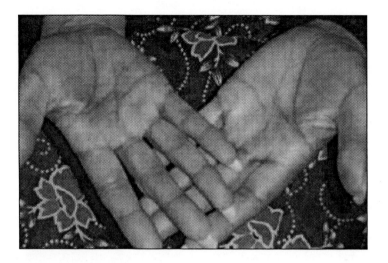

Then it got a bit worse.

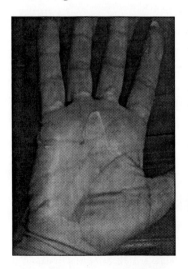 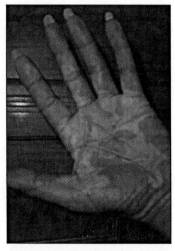

Then the blisters burst and the skin dried out. This had to be cut off. I could do my hands myself, but poor Rob got the job off cutting the stuff off my feet and then smothering them in moisturising lotion. I had to wear white cotton gloves and socks to keep everything clean, as the remaining skin was so thin. While preparing food I had to wear thin rubber gloves like the nurses wear. I was frightened that the skin would end up in someone's dinner! But there was a silver lining to this. All that horrid hard skin came off my feet and I was left with feet like a child just learning to walk. (That reminds me, if you have a child just learning to walk, please make sure the soles of their shoes are quite thick. Soft skin on hard stones hurts!)

With feet like this I often found it hard to walk. There was no pain, but have you ever tried walking on blisters? Not easy, is it? Then there was all that moisturising lotion – I did a lot of slipping about inside my shoes. And I started to have some fun…

July 7th, 2005. (I often wonder if the bombers chose that day so we could call it 7/7 without confusing the Americans.) No one told me until the day after that my sister Sarah worked in London two days a week. I had always thought she was in Reading. I called her. She hadn't been there that day – thankfully.

'I think I should stay away from London for a while,' I said.

'Oh, they won't do it again so soon, I'm sure.'

'It's not "them" I'm worried about, it's the English police.'

'What?'

'Well,' I told her, 'I'm wearing a headscarf and I've got a wire coming out of my t-shirt!' But she didn't think it was very funny.

Then there was the man who decided that I had parked my motor home too close to his car. Maybe I had, but that was no reason for him to yell at my son. Billy just told him to get into his car by the passenger door, and went back to his games console. By the time I arrived back, the guy was furious. He shouted and swore at me. I can't repeat what he said because I wasn't really listening. I was desperately trying to recall what it was that Sue had told me to say in these situations. Then I remembered. When the guy spluttered and ran out of words to shout I, very calmly, said, 'I really think that if getting into your car via the passenger door is all you have to worry about, then you should go home and think yourself bloody lucky!' Then I wobbled off with my slippery walk. With that, my headscarf, and the white gloves in the middle of summer, I guess he realised that I was a bit worse off than he was. Best part of it all was that while he was yelling at me, he had attracted quite a crowd of onlookers. He must have felt a right miserable git. I felt great!

There was also that happy trip to Tesco's – what fun that was! As I wobbled my way across the car park I noticed a flash car pull up and park in a disabled bay. The guy who got out of it looked as fit as a fiddle. I hate able-bodied people who park in these spaces, making some poor old or disabled person walk much further than necessary. So I managed to wobble my way into this guy's path as he left his car. He had no choice but to look at me. 'Oh,' I said, 'I really hope the day never comes when you actually *need* that space,' and then I wobbled off again. I have to say that he did look suitably embarrassed and that made me feel so good.

As I entered the shop I must have looked quite bad because a 'greeter' came to me and asked if I would like to use one of their disabled buggies. I didn't consider myself disabled, but there were plenty of spare buggies and it looked like fun. It was too, especially when I spotted a couple of friends and chased them around the shop. Ann will never forgive me for that! Still, it did give my feet a bit of a rest.

Another time I was in a hurry and needed to get some tomatoes, but it seemed that everyone else wanted tomatoes as well, I couldn't get near the box for ages. In the end I removed my gloves and stuck my hand out towards the little red fruits. Suddenly I was alone. No one wanted to go near any fruit or veg that I might have touched with those hands!

After that I would often whip my gloves off if I didn't want to stand in a queue as well. I would show everyone my hands and say, 'Excuse me, but my feet look like this too, does anyone mind if I push in the front?' Nobody ever did. Whether they felt sorry for me or just didn't want to look at me, I didn't care. The point was that I didn't waste time waiting in queues.

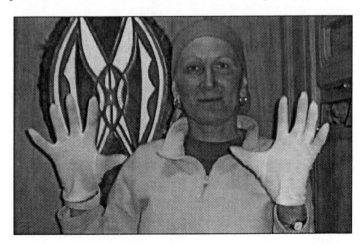

I had discovered that looking ill had plenty of advantages, and I used them to the full, embarrassing selfish people whenever I could.

But I found it hard to cope with all those sympathetic looks from people. I didn't want their sympathy. I wanted to forget the state I was in and just get on with life. I was able to do this with my friends Mandy and Clair, but so many others would not know how to talk to me. I had come across the same thing when our little boy had died and then, just like now, I had wanted to shout, 'Hey, I'm still the same person, I'm still me in here, you can still treat me the same!'

It was the people who assumed that I was going to die that really made me angry. There was *no way* I was going to die. Don't these people realise just how common breast cancer is? Just pick up any woman's magazine – they are always running stories about women with cancer.

Yes, I know that people do die of cancer, but a lot of people don't. Then, just as now, I knew that the cancer in me could be totally obliterated and still come back and kill me; but if it does that, then it's in for one hell of a fight. I've got a son who I need to see through his teens and into a good marriage, so I have no intention of going anywhere just yet.

Besides, I have said for years that I'm not going anywhere until my grandmother comes to get me, and I haven't seen either of my two wonderful grandmothers yet!

I started getting ill again. It wasn't as bad as when I had to go into hospital, but bad enough. I would have the energy to get up and make Billy some breakfast and see him off to school, but then I would have to go back to bed. It would take me all day to shower and take the dog for a walk because I had to keep stopping to sleep. In the evenings Billy and I would have to wait for Rob to come home from work and cook the dinner. I was just too exhausted to move by then. There were times when I just spent the day in bed. I was too tired to get up, too tired to cry about it. By now all my hair had completely gone. I had been told that the eyebrows and lashes would be the last to go and mine were thinning out nicely. My fingernails had split and fallen off and my toenails were starting to do the same. I felt like I was dropping to bits, but all the time I was grateful, because I knew that I was one of the lucky ones.

With the line in my chest I didn't have to have the needle for the chemo, I didn't have to sit there while a nurse tried time after time to get a needle into a vein that would simply collapse. I was never sick in public, I never cried with pain and I never got those awful headaches from wearing the cold cap! I wasn't lying terminally ill in that London hospital that the nurse had told me about – I knew that I would soon have an operation that would (hopefully) save my life. For many cancer-sufferers, surgery is not possible; it depends where the cancer is. For many chemotherapy is their only hope. Yes, I felt ill, but I also – always – felt so lucky.

I also felt lucky that it was only me with the cancer. I would look at my son and thank every god that anyone believed in that it wasn't him.

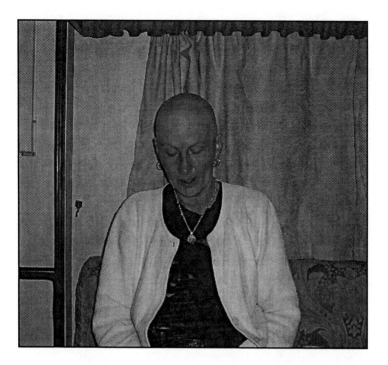

The last time I went for chemo was so hard. Rob and I had arrived early, I had had my blood taken, and we had gone to the restaurant for some lunch – but I couldn't eat. Instead I cried. I don't think Rob really knew what to do, but I just couldn't face going back upstairs for the chemo.

He managed to calm me down and get me up the stairs, but as we approached the door to the St Luke's wing I broke down again. Rob and the nurses were telling me that the worst was over, but I knew it wasn't. Chemo isn't like any other medicine at all. The body does not get used to it. It does not get easier, it just gets harder. I knew I was ill, yet I had to let some-one fill my body with drugs that were going to make me feel a lot worse. It was that I couldn't face. Eventually Rob managed to persuade me to go in and, as I sat in the chair waiting for my treatment, I realised that I didn't have the energy to get up and leave. At one point a nurse came and gave me a prescription for the pills I needed to keep the skin on my hands and feet. Usually I would have to go to the pharmacy and fetch them myself, but one look at me told the nurse that someone else would have to do it. She was afraid I might not come back.

Of course, I did have that last treatment; I did have the pump attached as usual afterwards; and I did leave with the next two pumps in my bag.

The next two weeks were a blur – I think I slept most of the time. That last pump was hard to put on too. In fact, I almost didn't do it. As usual I unhooked it to have a shower (I could only ever do this once a week, other days the pump had to hang on a special hook and I would have to wash myself around the line). After I had dried myself off I picked up the new pump. I had it in my hand and just looked at it for ages. I just didn't want to put it on. It crossed my mind that I could smash it and claim that I dropped it, but what would be the point in that? Rob would only take me back to St Luke's for another and the NHS would only have to pay for it again. I sat on the bathroom floor, my head leaning on the shower door, and sobbed. I had seen people at St Luke's crying and saying that they didn't know why. I knew why.

I didn't put the pump on straight away. I have to admit that I just couldn't do it. Instead I went back to bed and slept until about two thirty in the afternoon. It was lovely, I felt so free. There was no bag around my waist to get in the way when I turned over. I had taped the line to my belly, so even that didn't get in my way and, for the first time in six months, I was able to sleep on my front.

I had to put the pump back on eventually. I did it just before Billy came home from school.

One week later it came off again and I didn't have to put another one on. It was Tuesday 27th September, two days before my forty-fifth birthday – and it was the best birthday present I have ever had. I remember dropping the pump into that little yellow box the hospital had given me and feeling that I would soon be free. I had been told that the chemo would take about two weeks to leave my system and I couldn't wait to start feeling better again.

It was a week later that I weighed myself. My size eight jeans were held up by a belt and flapping about around my knees. I knew I'd lost weight, but I had only wanted to drop a dress size, not turn into Victoria Beckham! I had been a twelve at the start of treatment. I'm not going to say how much I weighed that day, but it was under seven stone. At first it was a nice feeling, being the weight I was at sixteen, and I had this crazy idea that I should find my old school uniform and try it on. Then I looked in the mirror. Yuck! Collar bones and hips all jutting out, ribs on display. That might be all very well for some silly pop or TV star, but I didn't want to look like a malnourished stick insect! I think a nice juicy steak is called for, I thought, with plenty of chips and a couple of big duck eggs. Then my stomach started to shift. OK, maybe a nice roast dinner, with plenty of crispy potatoes. It shifted some more and I pushed away all thoughts of a good fried breakfast and headed for the Fortisip again. Maybe next week!

Soon I was feeling a lot better; it's quite amazing how quickly a person can recover from chemo. It seemed that as soon as it was out of my system I was back to normal. Then I had to see Mr Laidlaw again – about the operation.

Part Three

In Hospital

This time I decided to give Mr Laidlaw the benefit of the doubt. I had thought that I hated him, but maybe that was just because he had been the one who had to tell me I had cancer in the first place. He had also been the one who had to tell me I was going to lose my hair. I thought there was a chance that he could actually be a nice person, it's just that he has a rotten job sometimes. I was right.

At this appointment he explained the operation to me. He had told me months before that I would need a mastectomy and that there was a possibility I could have a reconstruction done at the same time. Now he told me that he was going to cut under my arm, remove my left breast, move a muscle from my back and put it in my front and fill up the gap with a plastic thing that could be pumped up. The only thing I was interested in was what I would look like after the op.

I have never been the prettiest of women and have always felt that my boobs were my best feature. I was known for wearing bras that 'shoved 'em up and out' and for arranging my cleavage under the nose of any man to get what I wanted. There was no way I was going to let a simple thing like a mastectomy stop me from doing that.

The two breast care nurses, Sue and Pauline, showed me loads of photos of others who had undergone the same operation. Most of them looked quite good. I decided that as long as I wore a good bra, then I could look OK. I was just a little disappointed at the thought of never wearing my strappy little summer tops again. For some reason I thought I might be left with scars on my chest, but Mr Laidlaw assured me that I wouldn't. 'I'm going to cut you under here,' he said, running his finger down my side. 'From under your arm to about here' – just under my breast. 'You may have a scar on your back, but that depends on how your skin reacts. I will try not to cut there. The only scar you should have on the front is where I take the nipple away. And you can always have another one tattooed on later. They are very good actually, very realistic.'

I was beginning to like this man after all. I decided that a scar on my back wouldn't be too bad. I could always say I had been bitten by a shark – while surfing in a competition – somewhere off Hawaii, of course.

Everyone kept asking me, 'Are you sure this is what you want?' Yes, of course it was. The mastectomy was essential for my life, and the reconstruction was essential for my sanity. I know that many women don't bother with a reconstruction. I know that many just can't be bothered, or can't face it, or just don't care. I even know one woman who has had both boobs off, no reconstruction, and wears a special bra. She looks great and even goes swimming. If you hadn't been told, you would never guess that she was flat-chested; but I knew that I wouldn't be able to cope with that. For me personally, a reconstruction at the same time as the mastectomy was vitally important. Every woman is different – if you ever have that decision to make, make it alone. It's your body, your choice, and if someone else doesn't like your decision, well – tough.

My mother once asked me, 'Why are you bothering with a reconstruction at your age?'

Excuse me! What age? I was only forty-four. At what age am I supposed to stop wanting to look good? At what age am I supposed to stop wanting to feel sexy? I told myself that she had only said that out of shock. After all, I was almost at the end of my chemo by then and I had only just told her I had cancer! I had tried to get away without telling her. There just didn't seem any point in worrying her – after all, I always knew I was going to get better.

On October 17th I went into hospital. I had been sitting on the bed I had been allocated for about three minutes when Pauline came to see me. She explained what would happen while I was there and told me to yell if I needed anything. After she had left a nurse came and introduced herself. She said she would be looking after me over the next few days. Still people kept asking me if I was OK about this operation. I didn't understand the fuss. After all, Mr Laidlaw seemed very confident and if there was going to be a problem it was going to be his problem – not mine. What did I have to worry about? All I had to do was go to sleep! No, operations have never bothered me at all.

I spent the rest of that day getting to know the other people in the bay (the ward was split into sections known as bays) and was pleased to find that they were a nice bunch of ladies.

From eight o'clock that night I wasn't allowed to eat

anything, but that was fine by me – I had seen the hospital food! At twelve o'clock on Tuesday 18th October I went into theatre. A nurse wheeled me down on my bed and I was left in a small room with three young lads who seemed intent on making me laugh. They succeeded quite easily because I wasn't nervous at all. Then Mr Laidlaw came in, drew on my back and went out again. The next person to enter the small room was the guy who stuck the needle in my arm, the anaesthetist.

I remember waking up, briefly, in the recovery room and looking at the clock. It was seven thirty and I was being sick! Then I was being taken back to the ward (apparently it was nine thirty by then) and I saw that Billy and Rob were there. I wondered if it was really a good idea for Billy to see me in that state – and the next thing I knew it was Wednesday morning.

I realised that I was lying in bed with nothing on except a squash top or compression vest – this is a vest tight enough to hug the body and prevent lumps and bumps forming after something has been removed from inside – which Pauline had warned me about, and I needed to go to the loo. I couldn't have got out of bed anyway, because there seemed to be rather a lot of tubes coming out of me. When the nurse came she remarked that I hadn't pushed the button. Button? Was there a button somewhere I should know about? What was it for? Oh, yes, I had been told. It was morphine for the pain, but, surprisingly enough, there was no pain. They must have given me something good in the theatre or the recovery room. After that it seemed that the same nurse was always standing there telling me that I should push the button for a pain-killer. I did once, just to get her to go away, and I soon started to feel a bit sick. I didn't push it again.

Later, I realised that the nurse had been checking on me and had, in fact, been going away again because suddenly it was about three o'clock in the afternoon and I was wide awake. I managed to convince the nurses that I wasn't in any pain and didn't need the morphine so they disconnected it and told me I could take pain-killing pills instead. Once I'd taken them, the oxygen tube was removed from my nose and I was able to get out of bed.

Pauline came to see me. She said that the operation had gone very well, but that I had spent a couple of hours in recovery because I was sick several times. It began to dawn on me then that it might have been the morphine causing the sickness. I'd only ever had it once before, when my first son Billy was born, and I was sick then too. Pauline then told me that I had been given two pints of blood. This didn't mean a lot to me but she went on to explain that it was rather a lot of blood for someone of my size to lose, so they had needed to replace it. Had it been Mr Laidlaw losing two pints it really wouldn't have mattered. Yes, I could see her point – the man was about twice my size, plus some.

When Pauline left, a nurse told me about the drains. Pauline had already warned me there could be up to four of these pipes coming out from my side, to drain away the excess fluid that the body makes in these circumstances. And there were four! Four tubes coming out of my side – four tubes with little boxes on the end that were filling up with a watery blood. They were to stay there for several days. Great, how was I going to get about with them hanging off me? The nurse took one of my pillows and removed the cover. 'Put them in this,' she said. Yes! Now I could move.

Five minutes later I was sitting in the sun outside the front of the hospital. I'm still not sure if I was supposed to go outside so soon after the operation, but it was a lovely, sunny day and it seemed such a shame to be stuck inside. (OK, so I wanted a smoke, but I wasn't going to boast about that on the cancer ward, was I?)

I wasn't the only one out there with a bald head and a packet of smokes, there were several of us. Sometimes we would go into one of the little gardens and sometimes we would sit outside the front door to the main building – it depended where the sun was. In my case, it also depended where Minnie was. That wasn't her real name of course. If I were to mention her real name she would be on my back with a solicitor faster than I could say, 'It wasn't me.' She was known as 'Moaning Minnie' so that's what I will call her. I didn't meet her on that first day – she was probably still in bed complaining about the pain, or the surgeon, or the pills, or something. I met her a few days later and wished I hadn't!

Those first few days in hospital were actually quite nice. It was lovely to have nothing to do but watch TV, sleep or struggle with a Sudoku puzzle. It was nice to have someone make my bed, clean up around me and cook my food. Well, at least they said they cooked it, sometimes I wondered. At least the salads were always warm!

The staff on ward F7 were lovely. The nurses were fantastic and the lady who served the food always had a smile on her face. Even the young lad who did the cleaning and served the cups of tea and coffee was charming, happy and nice to have around.

I spent a lot of time wandering around the hospital and met loads of people on different wards. When I got back I was usually told that I had just missed the doctors!

Mr Laidlaw came to see me on his rounds on the Wednesday evening. He wanted to see how well I was healing. Until that point I hadn't taken off my squash top and I hadn't seen what I looked like. I hadn't quite dared. Now I had to. Actually, I didn't have to. I was asked if I minded – but I figured that I was going to have to look at some point anyway. So I opened the zip and undid the hooks. What I saw was nowhere near as scary as I had thought it would be.

My nipple was gone and in its place was a thin line, the boob was flatter and a bit square, but that was about it. I was really pleased. I knew that the 'bag' inside the boob would be inflated at a later date to make the new breast the same size as my remaining boob – so the flatness didn't worry me. Mr Laidlaw seemed pleased with his work (and so he should be) and also pleased with the way I was healing. It was then that I noticed that I had no stitches. Not one! I had been glued back together. It looked a bit of a mess under my arm at that point, but I could clearly see how small and thin my scar was going to be. It was not going to be noticeable at all. I didn't have a scar on my back either, it hadn't been necessary to cut me there.

So no boasting about the fight with a shark then. Wow, who thought up this envelope surgery? Give that person a medal! Fantastic, my Christmas trip to Cuba was looking good after all.

I wasn't allowed into the shower on my own for a couple of days. I don't think I could have managed it anyway. I had taken to wearing my pyjama bottoms, but not the top. I couldn't get it over my head because my left side was a bit stiff, though surprisingly enough, there was no pain. I would wear the squash top and put on my dressing gown when I left the ward. Washing was easy as long as I only 'dabbed' the wounds with one of the special cloths that the nurses handed out, but I did have to have someone else to wash my back. It was several days before we got the surgeon's black ink marks off.

There was a woman in the bed next to mine, Marcia, who had undergone a mastectomy too; but she was happy not to have any sort of reconstruction. What she wasn't happy about was the fact that after her drains had been taken out she started to bleed quite badly, and had to have them put back in. Opposite her was Helen. Helen was young and recently married. She was in there to put on weight for her next operation. Naturally, the hospital food wasn't exactly doing her the world of good, so she had to have plenty of 'build up' drinks and a drip that carried something similar into her. I never found out what was wrong with Helen; I don't think anyone else did either. We were all just pleased when someone ruled out Crohn's disease.

Opposite my bed was Katie. Well into her eighties,

Katie was the sort of 'little old lady' that everyone loves. She had a kind of childish innocence about her that made her really sweet. She didn't say much, but she smiled a lot. She also 'exercised' on her bed at two o'clock in the morning and had me panicking in case she fell off it! Once, she took herself off for a walk when no one was looking. She had almost made it to the door before she was brought back – grinning from ear to ear and making a joke about needing to escape. Life on the ward was slow and relaxed. OK, it was boring, but it was a nice kind of boring.

After a couple of days I decided to see how well I could cope without the painkillers. I've never been one for pumping too many chemicals into my body and I hadn't exactly had any pain. The nurses weren't too happy about it, but said I could give it a go. I was told to ask if I changed my mind at any time and off I went downstairs for a smoke.

I discovered that day that there really wasn't any pain. I think I must have been numb, because it just didn't hurt, but I did get very stiff and I started taking the painkillers again to loosen things up a bit so that I could move about more easily. That was the day I met Minnie.

'What are you in for?' she asked from behind a cloud of smoke. Blimey, I thought I smoked a lot for someone with cancer, but Minnie would have four or five to my one, and she made that question sound as if we were in prison.

'Cancer,' I said.

'Thought so.'

'Yeah, the bald head's a bit of a give away, isn't it?'

She then told me that she had just had a cancer operation too, but apparently the surgeon didn't do a very good job and she had been left with an infection. She showed me the small wound left from her lumpectomy. It looked OK to me, but then what do I know? I told her she should probably keep it covered. She had problems with her drains too, after all she did have *two* of them. They were awful, they kept dripping everywhere and they hurt all the time, and she had to carry them around with her, and she couldn't sleep properly because the nurses kept waking her up, and no one had given her fresh water that day, and there was nothing on the telly…

I didn't bother finishing my cigarette, I just stubbed it out and went back upstairs. I don't do sympathy. I don't like taking it and I don't give it out. Especially when I feel I've been *told* to!

It turned out that she and I had been admitted to hospital on the same day. We had both had our operation on the following day, by the same surgeon. We had then both been returned to the same ward (thankfully different bays), where we were looked after by the same nurses and the same staff. We both had cancer, but I had just endured six months of intensive chemotherapy followed by an operation to rearrange my torso, while she had simply had a lump removed and might have to have chemo or radiotherapy. I was grateful to all the people who had worked together to try to keep me alive, while she hated them for doing things to her. She didn't trust any of them and didn't like any of them. It seemed that after the nurses entered her bay they underwent some sort of metamorphosis into hideous uncaring beasts who were only interested in themselves and drank tea all day. Doctors became monsters who shouted and swore, and cleaners and tea ladies just never appeared. I think they had the right idea.

The bay I was in had a window overlooking the front door of the hospital. It was just to the side of this that most people went to sit and have a smoke. This is not the best first impression for a hospital to give, but it is a sight seen at most. I started looking out of the window before venturing downstairs. If Minnie was out there I would head for the little garden in the quad, or go back to bed with my book. Of course, there were times when she would appear just as I turned away from the window, or after I had sat myself on the wall and lit up, but there were usually plenty of other people to talk to. There was the woman with Lupus (a form of skin Tuberculosis) who also had cancer and had just been told that she had about two years left to live. The only thing that worried her was that she wouldn't be around to see her daughter through her teens and that it would be her husband who would have to cope with the hormonal strops all by himself. There was a guy in a wheelchair because the cancer had ruined the bones in his hips, but who was worried about leaving his flat empty for so long. There was a guy who nipped out for a quick puff while visiting his dying father, and the young lad who came out to celebrate that his girlfriend had regained consciousness. There was even the girl who said, 'Oh mine's all self inflicted, don't worry about me,' because she was a drug addict. There was a constant stream of people coming and going who gave us pathetic looks as they thought, Poor things, let them smoke, they're going to die soon anyway; as well as several people I knew, who had never seen me without hair or scarf and weren't sure who I was. I would smile and say hello and they would wander off asking their partners, 'Who was that?'

One person told me that I was *not* to sneak up on people I knew and shout '*Boo!*' in their ears. Apparently it wasn't the fact that I made them jump that bothered them, it was turning around to be greeted by a shiny head, no eyebrows, and a dirty great grin! But it was fun!

You have to have some fun in life, no matter what it throws at you. Cancer is the pits – it hurts and it's frightening – but my attitude when bad things happen is to deal with it, and then get on with life. If I can have some fun along the way – then great. Life does throw some shit, but life is still what you make it, even when your toenails drop off, or your teeth fall out.

One day I had just had a shower and was sitting on the bed struggling with those awful hospital socks that are designed to stop DVT. I had managed to get one on and was trying to stretch the other over my left toes when I felt something give. 'Ouch, what was that?' I said, more to myself than anyone else, but a nurse had overheard and came to see what the problem was. She looked at my foot just as I managed to get the sock off again, and she saw what had happened.

'Eeeeugh!' she said as she backed away.

'It's OK, it doesn't hurt,' I said. Helen was looking over with a concerned look on her face, and Katie looked rather worried.

'Ooohh, sorry, but I hate toenails,' said the nurse,

with a shiver. This from a woman who sticks needles into people and cleans up all sorts of unimaginable messes. I held up the last of my toenails – it was no longer attached to the toe – and the nurse fled the room. Helen said it wasn't very nice to go threatening people with toenails, but Katie just laughed. So that was it. All the toenails were now gone. I just had bits of nails left on some of my fingers. I sat there and looked at my hands and feet. Not a pretty sight, but nails grow.

The following day I had no choice but to eat the hospital food. I was getting a bit fed up with chicken, but the café downstairs had run out of baked potatoes. You may remember that in the summer of 2005 it was the beginning of the bird flu scare. We hadn't had it in England, but no one seemed to be taking any chances. We had to order our meals the day before we ate them and when they arrived we had to guess what it was we had ordered. Once, I was sure I had ordered a ham salad, but when it came it was chicken. Then my minced beef and mashed potatoes turned out to be minced chicken and – something! My Lancashire hotpot turned into chicken stew. When my sausages became drumsticks I got the point. Chicken was selling cheap! Even so, should they really be giving it to me? My cancer was hormonal and what is it they shove into the chickens to make them lay more eggs? I didn't really want to know – after all, I had to eat the stuff!

So there I was, using my teeth to tear the skin off a drumstick to reveal the miniscule bit of meat underneath, when I bit on something hard. OK, so the meat was tough, but it shouldn't be that tough! I thought I must have bitten the bone, so I spat it out on to the side of my plate and immediately felt something was wrong inside my mouth. I put the tip of my tongue up to the right side of my gum and that's what I felt – gum – where there should have been a tooth. The blinking thing had fallen out! There it was, nestled nicely on a bit of limp lettuce.

I wasn't really worried about it falling out at first. I've had a problem with calcium in the past and most of my teeth are actually crowns, but this one was one of the teeth that was screwed into the gum, so it shouldn't have just fallen out. Later that night, when I was cleaning my teeth I had a good look at them in the mirror. I found that I could easily see which of the teeth were crowns because there seemed to be a gap between them and my gums. The next day I mentioned it to a doctor who told me that it was probably due to the chemo. Sometimes it could make the gums recede. He told me not to worry, 'because things would sort themselves out soon enough'. I have to admit that they did. I made a trip to the dentist a few weeks later and she put back the missing tooth. She told me that the rest of my teeth were fine and the gums looked healthy.

I think that meant I had the lot, just about every side effect that chemotherapy could throw up. I lost my hair, toenails and fingernails; I lost the skin on my hands and feet and almost lost my immune system; I got sick, lost two stone in weight, slept for days at a time and then lost teeth, but the thing is – the chemo had worked! It had shrunk my tumour from ten centimetres diameter to something small enough to operate on. The operation had saved my life – for now, at least – but it was the chemo that had made it possible. And Mr Ian Laidlaw, of course. After all, he did the operation.

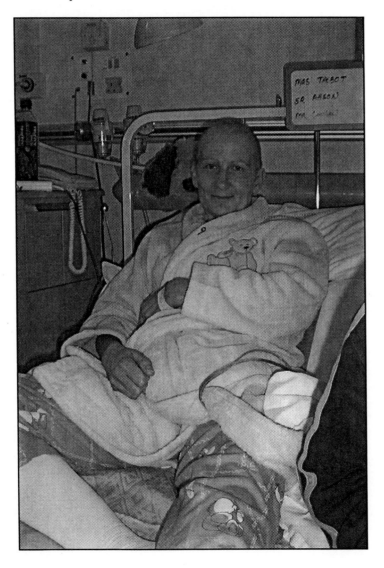

Part Four

After the Operation

Two weeks after the operation I was back at the hospital for the 'follow-up' appointment. This was a nightmare. The doctor I saw that day was the first horrible person I had met since this all began. Maybe she's a very good doctor, but she definitely needed to brush up on her people skills. If I never see her again it will be too soon.

I was nervous enough, going in to find out whether all the cancer had gone or not, without her attitude. I can remember her words as if she had said them just five minutes ago. I will remember them for the rest of my life. She sat at that desk, looking down at my notes as she spoke. Not once did she look up at me. She said, 'Right, it's not good. You only had a one-millimetre border of clear tissue, so the cancer is probably in your chest wall. Nine out of ten of your lymph nodes were infected, so it will be in your neck too. So you'll have to have radiotherapy. That will scar your lungs and could cause a heart attack...'

That's when I stopped listening. I stood up and stumbled out of the room with Rob following me. The very first person I saw in the waiting area was bloody Moaning Minnie.

'Hey, MJ,' she said, but I just turned and walked away from her. I felt that I had just been told that I had about six months left to live, and she was the very last person I wanted to have to listen to. Then Pauline appeared and guided me into a side room. 'Don't worry,' she said, 'I'll see to it that you don't have to talk to her, she won't get anywhere near you. Can I get you a drink?'

Yes, I thought, a large gin. But I didn't trust myself to speak.

Inside the small room I tried to tell Pauline what the doctor had said, but I was so upset that I couldn't seem to get the words out right. Rob just looked confused and a bit shocked. So Pauline went off to get Polly. I had met her a couple of times on the ward. One of Mr Laidlaw's team, Polly was tall, blonde and classy. She looks like the sort of woman I would usually hate (how dare she look that good?), but with her I just couldn't do it. Polly was just so nice I couldn't imagine anyone not liking her. (Tall, slim, blonde, pretty, and nice too – how dare she?) Polly doesn't talk to notes, she talks to people, and she looked at me as she spoke. She really only said what the other doctor had said, but she added things like 'could be' and 'maybe' and 'might be'. First she explained that a one millimetre border wasn't that bad, but it wasn't as good as they had hoped. So there was a 'slim' chance that the cancer could still be in the chest wall. Then she told me that I had nine lymph nodes – all of which had been removed and eight of which had been infected. So again, there was a slim chance it could have spread further into my neck.

Polly said that if the cancer was still in me it was too small to be detected, but they were not going to take any chances and I was being sent for radiotherapy to be on the safe side. I then asked about the scarring to my lungs and the risk of heart attack. I was told, 'When radiotherapy is given in this area there will be scarring to the left lung.' She drew a diagram on a piece of paper showing me just where the rays would be directed. I saw that it would just skim over the surface of the lung. 'But you won't know anything about that. It won't hurt and it won't affect you at all. The only time you'll know about it is if you ever have a chest X-ray and someone looks at it and says – "Oh, I see you've had radiotherapy."' That was a relief! Polly then went on to explain about this heart attack I had been told I was likely to have. It seems that ten or fifteen years down the line about one per cent of people who have had radiotherapy to the left breast do have heart attacks. It is believed that about one per cent of these attacks might be caused by the treatment. That was a relief too. She then told me that I couldn't start treatment yet anyway as my new boob had to be fully inflated first in case the skin got a bit damaged and decided to give up on any stretching. 'There's no great rush,' she said. 'Aren't you going on holiday soon? I told her, 'Yes, we were heading off to Cuba for two weeks on December 21st.'

'How fantastic, lucky you,' she said. 'Well, we don't want to risk you being ill on your holiday, so how about we start treatment when you get back?' That sounded good to me.

So, whereas I had left that other doctor's room be-lieving that I was either going to die of cancer or drop dead from a heart attack within about six months, I actually left the hospital feeling quite pleased with my results. Of course I was still at risk, but this was a risk I could cope with – for a few weeks anyway.

I saw Mr Laidlaw a couple more times before the year ended; to check how things were healing and to pump my new boob up. Everything was healing just fine and the mess under my arm was disappearing fast. In other words, the glue was coming off. The scar itself was hardly noticeable. At 'pump up' time I sat on the bed with my top off while Mr Laidlaw played about with a syringe. 'How exactly are you going to pump this up?' I asked.

'Oh, I could tell you,' he replied, grinning, 'but then I would have to kill you!' OK, so he didn't have his surgeon's head on that day!

He pushed the needle of the syringe into my back. I have no idea whereabouts because I couldn't feel a thing. I just watched as my left boob began to grow. Fascinating! But once I was 'pumped up' Mr Laidlaw noticed that something was not quite right. Somehow the bag inside had got twisted. We couldn't tell how twisted, of course, but it was obvious that something was wrong because I had a point sticking out right in the middle of my cleavage. It wasn't a big point, but it shouldn't have been there at all. 'I'm sorry, I don't like the look of that. I think I'm going to have to change it,' he said. He told me that it would be best to wait until everything had settled down again after the radiotherapy and that it would only mean a trip to day surgery. I didn't care, I was just happy to have my boobs back. As soon as my eight weeks were up I was going to get out of that squash top and into a bra and start enjoying life again.

It didn't quite work out as well as I had hoped. Not at first. A couple of days later I went shopping. I had tried on my old bras and bikini and found they didn't fit. It wasn't the size of the boob that was wrong, but I had lost so much weight. By now I had managed to get back up to eight stone and had no intention of gaining any more weight, so it wasn't surprising that my things didn't fit. First, I headed off to a good underwear shop and asked to be measured. I never buy bras without being measured, but this time I said I needed help because I had just had an operation. The woman knew what I was talking about so I was surprised at her reaction when she first saw my chest. 'How long ago did you have that done?' she asked.

'About six weeks ago.'

'You must have had it done at Frimley, then.'

I told her I had and she explained that it was one of the neatest jobs she had seen. 'They are always neat from Frimley,' she said. 'They always seem to do such a good job of it.'

It was then that I discovered that I wasn't quite right. Yes, I was the right size (almost) but I was the wrong shape and it was difficult to find a bra to fit both sides. My new left boob seemed to be further to the side than the right one. It was as if it was trying to escape under my arm. I ended up having to flatten the right side a bit just to keep things level and I still had to stuff the left. But I wasn't worried. I knew that I still wasn't 'finished' and hoped that when the bag inside was changed it would get better. At that point I was just looking forward to actually wearing a bra and going on holiday. First, I needed a bikini.

Have you ever tried to buy a swimsuit in the winter in this country? It's not easy is it? Why do shops only sell them in the summer? Do they think people don't swim in the winter, even in pools? I ended up at a specialist swimwear shop and had to pay almost £50. I had to get a size smaller than I usually wear. I had to flatten the right boob even more because it's not possible to go swimming with tissue stuffed down the bra. My 'point' would be on display too.

Oh, who cares? Who's going to look at a forty-five-year-old mother on the beach anyway, when there are bound to be plenty of younger girls?

While I was trying the bikini on, I noticed something. The marks from the drains were fading fast, but still visible. The two smaller ones were covered by the bikini, but the two larger ones were on display. What would be the funniest thing to say if someone asked about them? I decided on, 'Oh, I got them in Iraq,' and I would walk away and leave them to think all sorts of things!

The next stop was the dress shop. I wanted something nice and slinky for the evenings. Every woman on telly seemed to be wearing a particular style of dress that just about covered enough to make them respectable. I wanted something similar, but I was a little early. It seemed that everything I tried on had straps in strange places (if they had straps at all) and couldn't be worn with a bra. This is not good when one boob stays up and one sags!

I gave up, but on the way out of the shop I spotted

something. It was one of those dresses where the top is just two strips of material that come down from the neck to just cover the nipples before attaching themselves to the waistband. Knowing I couldn't possibly wear it, I tried it on. Apart from that point sticking out, the left side looked great. The right side didn't though. Maybe I would have that operation to lift up the right boob after all.

Our trip to Cuba that Christmas was fantastic, but that's another story. I'm not going to say too much about it here. I'll only tell you the bits that are connected to the cancer. The first problem I had was when I unpacked my case and couldn't find my wigs.

Before we had left I had washed, conditioned and dried them, wrapped them in a bag and put them in my case. I *know* I did. Billy even saw me do it, but neither of them were there when I opened it up. I hadn't travelled with a wig on. I hardly wore one anyway and a gnome-type Christmas hat had seemed easier to cope with on the plane. My hair was beginning to grow back, but it was still so short that I had wanted the wigs for evening wear, but I just had to go without. I admit to not feeling 'quite right' in a nice evening dress with hardly any hair. No one else seemed to notice, except one little girl who informed me that I looked like a man. I had to laugh at that because she was an ugly little thing and at least my hair would grow! She had also called an elderly lady 'lizard face' and none of the other kids liked her so I didn't feel too bad.

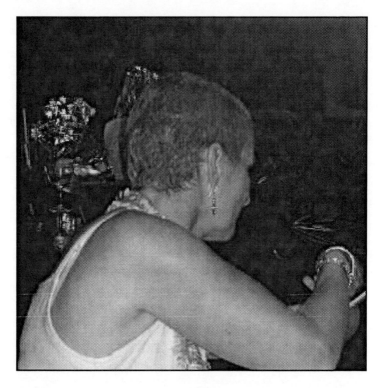

Sunbathing caused a small problem. Lying on my back on the sun beds was fine, but lying on my front wasn't so easy. I was so used to boobs that moved that I didn't think, and just turned over to toast my back. That was when I discovered that I could no longer lie flat on my front. Well, actually, I have never been able to lie flat on my front for very long because my boobs aren't small enough, but they did used to move and flatten out a bit. Now, of course, one of them wouldn't. I tried keeping my left arm bent up to offer a bit of support, but that just made my arm ache. It wasn't comfortable at all.

The beach was better. If I put my towel down on the sand, I found I could punch a small dip with my fist to put my left boob into. That way I could lie flat and tan my back, and I didn't have to wander about the beach looking for an empty sun bed or worry that someone would pinch it if I went for a swim.

I also discovered that swimming in the sea was better than in the pool. I'm not much of a swimmer anyway and the salt in the sea makes floating easier, so there isn't so much effort. This puts less strain on the left side.

One day we went to swim with dolphins. That was the day I learnt what the Americans mean when they say something is 'totally awesome'. We were told that we would be in the water for about an hour, so I used a life jacket. It was nice; I spent the time just bobbing about instead of having to tread water. I know, now, that if I hadn't had that jacket on I wouldn't have been able to stay in the water for so long and would have missed some vital moments with these beautiful creatures.

It was on Boxing Day that I had my worst problem. We had spent Christmas day visiting different places and heading up the mountains and into the rainforest. Some of the trip was done on the back of an old Russian army truck. Not only did the truck have no suspension, but it had a very high back. This was great for the view, but not so good if you had to haul yourself up and down using your arms to keep you steady. My left arm was getting tired and weak by the end of the day.

A rest in a mountain hotel helped and, by the next

day, I thought everything was going to be fine. It almost was. We spent that day trekking through the rainforest and learning about the wildlife and coffee growing. Then we came to the waterfall. At the waterfall our group split into two. One half took all the bags and carried on along that path, while the other half stripped off to hats and swimsuits and climbed into the waterfall. Guess which group we were in!

The water was cold to begin with, but we soon got used to it. We weren't just going to have a swim; we were going to climb down the waterfall. It was great. We spent the next hour or so slipping and sliding over rocks, jumping into the water and climbing out again as we made our way down. There was a lot of stretching to reach rocks and a lot of slipping when we missed. We had to follow the guide very carefully and do exactly as he said, but he made it look so easy and he was barefoot. We had running shoes on and probably looked like a group of drunks. At the bottom of the waterfall the only way back to dry land was to jump into a small lagoon and swim across it. I was one of the first in and started swimming to get out of the way of the others. I really didn't want a thirteen-stone bloke landing on top of me.

I got halfway across the lagoon when something happened. I have no idea what it was, but it hurt. The only way I can describe it is to say that it felt like cramp in the left side of my chest. Suddenly my left arm twisted up almost into the foetal position, my body jerked to the left and my face went under the water. For a second or two I couldn't move, but then everything started to loosen up again and I was able to kick my feet to get them underneath me and bring my face up out of the water again. Luckily, Rob had seen what had happened and came to help me out. He dragged me to the jetty and helped to get me up the ladder with the minimum of fuss. I don't think anyone even noticed. As I dried off and got dressed the pain started to fade and, by the time we were ready to leave, I was back to normal. I think it was the stretching and swimming that did it. I'm told that swimming uses almost every muscle in the body so maybe that one in my chest had thought it was still in my back and had not been sure how to react. It had felt like a cramp in the whole of my left side. I guess the muscle panicked!

The only other problem I had was when one woman did notice what had happened to me. I was at the pool bar and had reached out my left arm to pick up my drink. The woman must have noticed either my scar or the marks left by the drains – you had to be quite close to see either of them.

'I think you're very brave,' she said.

'Pardon?'

'Well, you've obviously had a little bit of a problem,' she was almost whispering, 'and I think you are very brave.'

This annoyed me. So I told her, 'Actually it wasn't a "little bit of a problem", it was a ruddy great big one. And there's nothing brave about wanting to stay alive!' and I left it at that. No one asked me about the marks from the drains, and I never did get to say, 'Oh, I got them in Iraq.'

Part Five

The Final Hurdle

The three of us arrived back from Cuba in the New Year with wonderful suntans and a new lease of life; but Rob had to go back to work, Billy had to go back to school, and I had to go back to treatment.

Back at St Luke's I was measured up for the radiotherapy machine and told exactly what would happen. I was advised to use an aqua cream for washing with while having treatment as it has nothing that dries the skin and no chemicals to react with the treatment. I soon discovered that it cleans well and leaves the skin feeling moisturised and soft. I still use it today. Again, everyone kept asking me if I was happy to have radiotherapy – if I was sure I wanted to go ahead with treatment. I suppose they have to keep asking, but with me it wasn't necessary. Of course I wanted to go ahead. If there was any chance that there was still some cancer in my body then I wanted it out – and as soon as possible please. Anyway, after chemo, radiotherapy was going to be a doddle!

The worst thing about radiotherapy is the time it takes out of the day. We were living in Cobham at the time, but Billy was at school in Farnborough. So, every day for six weeks, I would drive twenty-five miles to get Billy to school, and then drive to Guildford.

At St Luke's I would check in, then go into one of the little side rooms and strip off to the waist. Then, after donning one of those incredibly unsexy hospital gowns, I would wander over to sit in the waiting area. My appointments were all at nine forty in the morning. At that time of the day everything was usually still running to schedule. I think during the whole six weeks I was only late in twice. Every other time I was either called in bang on time or even early. I lay back on the table and put my left arm up to be tied to a small 'shelf'. It had to be tied to keep it still. After three minutes of treatment I was off again: heading back to Farnborough to walk the dog and start my day two or three hours late. The treatment itself only had one side effect – it made me tired. But then all that driving didn't exactly help.

I was fine for the first three weeks and then it hit me. I couldn't sleep during the day as I had too much to do, so by the evenings I was about finished. Cooking and washing up was the last thing I wanted to do. Thank heavens for microwave dinners! Normally I hate those things and I know that the lack of real food was not helping my energy levels, but it had to be done. Billy was in seventh heaven, as we were having pizza two or three times a week.

I was glad it was winter though, because the treatment did leave what looked like dirty marks on my breast and neck. At least I could cover them up with a polo-necked jumper.

Just after I started treatment I spotted Sue at work. Her hair looked different. 'Hey Sue,' I said, 'you've had your hair done, it looks good.'

'Thanks,' she said, putting a hand up to her hair – but she didn't do it right, she didn't pat it with pride. I saw how her hands touched the side of her head and I knew. Unconsciously she was checking it was still in place. Sue was wearing a wig.

For six months that woman had been worrying about me. For all that time she had been asking me how I was doing and insisting that she was doing great and getting better, but she wasn't. Her chemo pills hadn't worked and she was back on the hard stuff. I prayed that she would be OK, but over the next couple of weeks I knew my prayers were going to go unanswered.

As I was being treated for a cancer that only might still be there, Sue was being treated for a cancer that was taking over her body. Only a couple of people at the centre knew she was ill. Sue didn't like to talk about herself much; she was more concerned with the children she worked with and helping them to have fun. So I felt I couldn't ask her much about herself, but I watched as she became thinner and more tired-looking.

Then, one day, she called me and asked me to go in and see her. We sat in the kitchen of the community centre and, over a cup of caffeine-free tea, Sue told me what to do if things got really bad. She gave me doctors' names and telephone numbers to ring. She told me of some sort of test being held that might give seriously ill cancer patients some extra time. Sue was too ill for these tests, but she wanted to make sure that I would have the chance, if the cancer was still in my body. I couldn't take in a lot of what she said, I just kept looking at her and thinking, What a wonderfully thoughtful person. She must have been a fantastic mother. There she was, knowing she didn't have much time left, but she was thinking of me. Sue knew she was dying; yet still, she was putting other people first.

Just a week later I was asked to go to the office and have a word with Val. One look at Val's face told me what she was going to say. Sue Crane – the world is a sadder place without you in it.

About this time I got a phone call from Pauline. Apparently a national newspaper was doing a piece on Frimley Park Hospital and cancer treatment. They wanted to interview someone who had received this new 'envelope surgery', and wanted to know if I would mind being that someone. This was the first time I had heard the word 'new' in connection with envelope surgery. Until then, I had thought that the operation I had was common practice. I had no idea that it was quite new and not many people had received it. I felt quite proud. And, of course, I was happy to be interviewed by the paper and happy to tell the country how great I think Frimley Park really is.

I was interviewed over the phone and then, a couple of weeks later a woman came to St Luke's to meet me and take some photographs. I had been told that they would send me a copy of the article before they published it to see that I approved – but they never did. One day – after treatment had finished – I got a call at about five o'clock to say that I was going to be in the paper the next day. I went straight to the computer and emailed all my friends and rang my mother. I wanted everyone to see my little bit of fame.

As is typical with newspapers, they got everything wrong. The article stated that I was diagnosed in February when actually it was April; they said I had my operation in June, when actually it was October. They also stated that I had six months of chemo before the op. This was true, but no matter how hard I try I cannot fit six months in the space between February and June! There were lots of little things like this that they got wrong, like saying it was my right breast when it was really my left, but never mind. The papers were also saying that there was a new drug that would save lives. They seemed to give the impression that it was definitely going to cure breast cancer and women all over the country were demanding it. The three doctors I asked all told me the same thing – that no one really knew if it was any better than the Tamoxafin that I was on. It was just a lot more expensive.

Mr Laidlaw's interview was quite good, though. It was interesting to read what he actually did to me, but I'm glad I didn't know that much before he did it!

The article did show Frimley Park in a positive light and said that I was very happy with the result of the operation – and that was the main thing. My mother rang that day and said, 'It's your picture, but who did they interview?'

Towards the end of my radiotherapy something happened. My body clock started ticking again. I was tired, I was feeling miserable a lot of the time, I cried at the smallest thing, and now this! I had been told that if my periods ever came back I was to tell a doctor straight away, so I mentioned it to one of the people doing the radiotherapy. The next day I was told that I had an appointment to see a doctor right after treatment. As soon as I was dressed I went upstairs.

I was told that I would need to have an injection every

twenty-eight days for about two years. This was because of the Tamoxafin that I had started to take. Tamoxafin is designed to prevent the return of breast cancer, but you can only take it if you have passed the menopause or else it can cause cancer of the womb. Chemo usually brings on the menopause and for six months I had thought it had done that to me too – but not so.

The injection works by controlling hormones and it kicks in straight away. I had the injection in the morning and by about five o'clock I was feeling great. My miserable feelings had gone, I was happy and when someone shouted at me for parking right where they had wanted to park I just grinned at them and walked away. No more periods, no more PMT, no hot flushes, and no more temper tantrums or depression – just instant menopause. Fantastic! It was another silver lining – actually, a gold lining!

When radiotherapy finished I had to have another mammogram and a scan. It wasn't so bad this time. At least I only had one boob to squash into that machine. 'I'll apologise now,' I told the nurse as I walked into the room, 'for any swearing I might do.'

She laughed. 'I'm used that that, don't worry,' she said.

Mammograms hurt. I can't wait for someone to invent a way of screening breasts without squashing them almost flat. The results were ready within a few minutes and I was told they looked clear. Then I went for the scan – at least that didn't hurt. The woman who did this was the same woman I had seen almost a year before for my biopsy. 'You're not going to stick needles into me today, are you?' I asked. She wasn't going to, it was just a scan. She said everything looked fine there too, except that my prosthesis was a little bit twisted, but we knew that anyway.

So everything had 'seemed' clear. I went home and hoped I wouldn't get a letter telling me otherwise. In these cases I believe that no news is good news. I didn't get a letter.

Then I had to wait for my skin to return to normal (it peeled like sunburn) before going back to see Mr Laidlaw about my prosthesis. I was looking forward to having it done. By now some of the feeling was coming back in my side and having a piece of plastic wrapped around my left side was beginning to get on my nerves. It ran under my skin just where a bra would go and whenever I stretched or moved too much I could feel it getting tight. I had given up wearing a bra because to make my boobs level I had to have one that was too small, and it was uncomfortable to have the right one flattened all the time. I had gone back to wearing the squash top for several weeks. Mind you, it was really comfortable. Never mind sports bras, I decided that when I went back to training I'd wear that squash top. Nothing moved under that and I never had to 'adjust' it no matter what I did.

The point from the fold in the prosthesis was beginning to aggravate my skin too and, although it didn't hurt, it wasn't exactly comfortable either. I hoped that the new gel-filled insert would be more comfortable and give me a better shape.

I had to see Dr Laing first and he explained again the importance of those monthly injections. He seemed to be almost apologising for it, but I was happy about it; those injections kept me calm and made me feel good. Then he told me that I would need a bone density scan. I had already been told that it is believed that chemo can cause osteoporosis, so this scan is just to keep an eye on things. I have been taking a bone drug and I take calcium tablets so I'm keeping my fingers crossed but I had suffered just about all the other side effects of the chemo – surely it could cut me some slack now and leave my bones alone!

Later that same day Mr Laidlaw told me that he couldn't change my prosthesis yet. He said I was still a bit swollen and my skin wasn't really back to normal. He knows more about these things than I do, so I thought I would just have to put up with things for a bit longer. I mentally went through my wardrobe looking for high-necked t-shirts and I hoped the summer wouldn't be too hot for that squash top. Then I noticed that Mr Laidlaw had a syringe in his hand. Apparently I was going to be pumped up again. Another tube of salty water was injected in and I watched once more as my boob grew. I had taken a bra with me to show how bad the prosthesis looked, and now I dug it out of my bag and tried it on.

It was much better. In fact, at first sight I thought the new boob might now be too big and that I would have to stuff the other cup of my bra to even up my cleavage. But not so.

I had been a D-cup before the cancer, but I had lost a lot of weight while on chemo and gone down to a C-cup. I had a C-cup bra with me, but when I got home I tried on a D-cup and it fitted even better. Fantastic! Not perfect, but the next best thing.

I have to have a small 'chicken fillet' insert on both sides – in the left to create a smooth slope upwards, and in the right to boost it up a bit – but once I'm dressed my chest looks great.

So the squash tops have been washed and put in my sports bag and my summer tops – that show off my cleavage – are ready to wear again. I don't care if the point of the prosthesis shows, no one should be looking that close anyway, and it won't be for long. Once the new prosthesis is put in I'll be completely free: free of that thing under my arm, free to go back to training, and free to get on with my life. I haven't decided yet if I'll have the right boob lifted to match the left, but it's highly possible that I will – eventually. As for having the nipple tattooed on – well, the only person to ever see it is Rob and he's not bothered, so is it really important? Maybe I'll think about it when the time is right.

Right now I'm just grateful. I'm grateful to Dr Laing, Mr Laidlaw and all the dozens of others who helped to keep me alive. I believe that I was given the very best treatment possible for my type of cancer – and by the nicest of people. Of course, I know that the cancer could still come back and kill me, but I also know that it's going to have one hell of a fight on its hands if it does!

Cancer is frightening. But it can be beaten. Chemotherapy is scary and very frightening. I hope that, one day, a simple pill or injection will be able to shrink any tumour and chemo can be relegated to medical museums. As chemo eats into the cancer it also eats into the body. It takes away the hair, nails, skin and so much more – but right now I think it's wonderful. It helped to save my life.

As I write this it is just over a year since I was first diagnosed. Then I was frightened, so very scared, but now I feel as if my life is beginning again. I've been given another chance and boy, am I going to use it!

And those silver linings? The skin on my feet is new and smooth – so much easier to care for. My hair is thicker stronger and more healthy – and curly. I've always wanted long curly hair! I've dropped a dress size. My periods have stopped with no hot flushes, fainting spells or emotional outbursts. And by the time I'm 'finished' I'll be able to throw away the scaffolding and buy the neat, pretty bras I wore twenty years ago because I'll have great new boobs.

But best of all, I'm alive!

Printed in the United Kingdom
by Lightning Source UK Ltd.
132488UK00001B/36/A